Homemade

A Complete Beginner's Guide to Natural DIY Cosmetics you can Make Today

Jane Aniston

Introduction

I want to thank you for choosing to download the book, "*Homemade Makeup — A Complete Beginner's Guide to Natural DIY Cosmetics You Can Make Today.*"

This book contains all the information you need to know in order to start making your own natural, chemical-free makeup at home today. The ingredients used to make these cosmetics are cheap and easily available and the process of making them couldn't be simpler!

In this book, we'll cover the differences between homemade cosmetics and the store-bought variety. In addition, I'll show you why you really should ditch the expensive, toxin-filled store-bought variety and start making your own natural, healthy, chemical-free alternatives at home.

This book also includes 28 natural makeup recipes covering all of the various cosmetics you use in your daily life. Each recipe will list the ingredients required to make the makeup and then guide you through the process of exactly what you'll need to do, with simple, easy-to-follow step-by-step instructions, meaning you can be making your own cosmetics in no time at all!

Once you see how fantastic natural homemade makeup is, you'll never want to go back to the harmful, store-bought variety, which can be toxic to not only your body but also the environment.

Thank you again for downloading this book. I hope you enjoy it!

Jane Aniston

© **Copyright 2015 by Eddington Publishing - All rights reserved.**

This document is geared towards providing exact and reliable information in regards to the topic and issue covered. The publication is sold with the idea that the publisher is not required to render accounting, officially permitted, or otherwise, qualified services. If advice is necessary, legal or professional, a practiced individual in the profession should be ordered.

- From a Declaration of Principles which was accepted and approved equally by a Committee of the American Bar Association and a Committee of Publishers and Associations.

In no way is it legal to reproduce, duplicate, or transmit any part of this document in either electronic means or in printed format. Recording of this publication is strictly prohibited and any storage of this document is not allowed unless with written permission from the publisher. All rights reserved.

The information provided herein is stated to be truthful and consistent, in that any liability, in terms of inattention or otherwise, by any usage or abuse of any policies, processes, or directions contained within is the solitary and utter responsibility of the recipient reader. Under no circumstances will any legal responsibility or blame be held against the publisher for any reparation, damages, or monetary loss due to the information herein, either directly or indirectly.

Respective authors own all copyrights not held by the publisher.

The information herein is offered for informational purposes solely, and is universal as so. The presentation of the information is without contract or any type of guarantee assurance.

The trademarks that are used are without any consent, and the publication of the trademark is without permission or backing by the trademark owner. All trademarks and brands within this book are for clarifying purposes only and are the owned by the owners themselves, not affiliated with this document.

Table of contents

Chapter 1: Why you should stop using store-bought makeup and start making your own at home!

Chapter 2: Insider Tips On Creating Your Own Cosmetics

Chapter 3: Natural Makeup Recipes – Face

    1. *Simple Soothing Makeup Base*

    2. *Oil-Control Makeup Base*

    3. *Powder Foundation for Normal Skin*

    4. *Powder Foundation for Dry Skin*

    5. *Powder Foundation for Oily Skin*

    6. *Liquid Foundation for Normal Skin*

    7. *Liquid Foundation for Dry Skin*

    8. *Liquid Foundation for Oily Skin*

    9. *Blemish Control Concealer*

    10. *Simple Flush Blusher*

11. Raspberry Crush Blusher

12. Hibiscus Blusher

13. Contour Powder

14. Simple Bronzing Powder

15. Silky Smooth Finishing Powder

16. Oil Control Finishing Powder

Chapter 4: Natural Makeup Recipes – Eyes

17. Cream Eye Shadow

18. Powder Eye shadow

19. Natural Cream Eyeliner (Black)

20. Natural Cream Eyeliner (Brown)

21. Natural Mascara (Black)

22. Natural Mascara (Brown)

Chapter 5: Natural Makeup Recipes – Lips

23. Easy Glide Lipstick (Red)

24. Easy Glide Lipstick (Nude)

25. *Matte Lipstick (Red)*

26. *Matte Lipstick (Tan)*

27. *Glossy Lipstick (Red)*

28. *Glossy Lipstick (Nude)*

Conclusion

A message from the author, Jane Aniston

FREE BONUS!

As a free bonus, I've included a preview of one of my other best-selling books, "Homemade Makeup - A Complete Beginner's Guide to Natural DIY Cosmetics You Can Make Today" - Includes 28 Organic Makeup Recipes! Scroll to the end of this book to read it.

ALSO…

be sure to check out my other books. Scroll to the back of this book for a list of other books written by me along with download links!

Chapter 1

Why you should stop using store-bought makeup and start making your own at home!

Makeup is something most women simply can't live without. Some women, in their search for beauty, have even gone as far getting permanent cosmetics tattooed on their faces (permanent eyebrows, for example). Personally, I see nothing wrong with wanting to look your best, but at the end of the day, one question we need to ask ourselves is: "What exactly are the ingredients in my beauty products?"

With almost all cosmetics containing numerous chemical ingredients, it can be a bit unsettling to think about the potential long-term effects these ingredients could be having on our bodies. Behind the glamour of the cosmetics industry, there's always the danger that the products we think are safe to put on our skin, might in actuality not be as safe as we think.

After studying the cosmetics industry, the truth is that these products have some of the largest mark-ups of any you're likely to find on the high street or in the mall! Your favorite face cream that cost you $80 may well have only cost as little as $2 to make, while that trendy lipstick you paid $30 of your hard-earned money for may actually only have a monetary value of $0.75! If you've bought thousands of dollars worth of cosmetics over the years, this realization can be pretty depressing. It doesn't feel good to know that all this time we've been duped by the cosmetics industry via slick marketing campaigns, while they made massive profits out of us unsuspecting consumers.

This is certainly something I've been a victim of. In the past, one of the things I would regularly spend money on was a good (and very expensive!) lipstick. Whenever I was having a bad day, I would head down to my favorite store and treat myself to a new shade. My friends would easily be able to tell if I was having a good year or not by the number of lipsticks I had in my collection! In hindsight, knowing what I know now, I feel a real sense of regret that I didn't get around to making my own cosmetics earlier. If I had of done, my bank balance certainly would have been a little healthier, and that money could have been better put to use.

The thing about the cosmetics industry is that even if you have a suspicion you're being ripped-off, it just feels that buying these products is something you *have to do*. I know a lot of women who would gladly fork over an inordinate amount of money for an excellent foundation! Why? Because you simply can't put a price on the confidence that looking your best can give you. The marketing used to sell cosmetic products has preyed on the insecurities of women for far too long. We are constantly bombarded with the message that if you want to feel good about yourself you need to look like a cover model; the implication being that the only way you'll be able to do that is to use their (expensive!) cosmetics. It's even gotten to the point where some women consider certain brands of makeup to be status symbols, much like they may do with a pair of expensive shoes or a designer handbag.

Am I immune to the marketing hype surrounding cosmetics? Honestly, no. I confess that even after learning the heartbreaking truth about the beauty industry I still get excited when I'm in the store browsing the makeup department. I still look at each lipstick color and eye shadow shade and imagine how I would incorporate them to achieve all sorts of glamorous looks. The only difference now is I don't purchase anywhere near as many products as I used to. These days I usually just look around in search of color inspiration, make a mental note and then create my own cosmetics at home. If you're thinking that the only reason I do this is to save a few dollars, you're wrong. Unfortunately there's more to it than that.

Harmful Ingredients Abound!

One of the sad realities when it comes to cosmetics is that the vast majority contain toxic ingredients. Even makeup products labeled as "all-natural" often times contain ingredients that may increase susceptibility to skin allergies, cancer, infertility and reproductive problems. If you're not sure about which ingredients you'd be best to avoid, here's a list of chemical nasties which are often used in cosmetics. Considering that human skin absorbs almost 60% of what is applied to it, this list will make you think twice next time you're about to splurge on expensive cosmetics.

- **Coal Tar** – Although already banned in the EU and Southeast Asia, there are still some products being sold in the US that contain this carcinogen. It's often found in treatments for dry skin as well as in anti-dandruff shampoos. Coal tar is also known as FD&C Red No.6.

- **Ethoxylated surfactants and 1,4-dioxane** – Created when carcinogenic ethylene oxide is added to a cocktail of other chemicals. This nasty toxin is found in some cosmetics, and unfortunately, is commonly found in baby washes being sold in the US. As a general rule, if you want to err on the safe side, avoid ingredients that contain the syllable "eth".

- **DEA/TEA/MEA** – These chemicals are used as foaming agents for body washes, soaps, and shampoos. All are suspected of being potential carcinogens.

- **Fragrance/"Parfum"** – A catchall for unknown chemicals like phthalates. Fragrance has been proven to cause dizziness, headaches, asthma, and even allergic reactions in some unsuspecting victims.

- **Formaldehyde** – A proven irritant and likely carcinogen that can be found in hair dye, nail products, and shampoos. It is already banned in the EU.

- **Lead** – A carcinogenic contaminant found in most lipsticks and hair dyes. Since it's not officially considered to be an ingredient, you'll never see this listed on any beauty product.

- **Hydroquinone** – An ingredient used to peal and lighten skin. It is banned in the UK due to the fact it's been linked to cancer and reproductive disorders.

- **Mineral oil** – This petroleum byproduct can be found in moisturizers, baby oils, and styling gels.

- **Mercury** – An allergen that is known to impair brain function and development. Can be found in select eye drops and mascaras.

- **Parabens** – Used to preserve ingredients in many beauty and baby products. Has been linked to cancer, reproductive disorders, and endocrine problems.

- **Oxybenzone** – A chemical sunscreen that accumulates in fat cells. It can cause allergic reactions and hormone irregularity.

- **Phthalates** – A type of plasticizer that is banned in the EU and just recently, in California. It can be found in perfumes, deodorants, and lotions; and has been linked to kidney, liver, and lung damage.

- **Paraphenylenediamine (PPD)** – Present in hair dyes and styling products. Proven to be toxic to skin and can cause complications with the immune system.

- **Silicone derived emollients** – An ingredient added to some cosmetic products to make them feel soft. It has been linked to skin irritation and tumor enlargement.

- **Talc** – Has a similar composition to asbestos. Can be found in some blushes, eye shadows, baby powders, and deodorants. Has been linked to respiratory problems and ovarian cancer.

- **Sodium lauryl (ether) sulphate (SLS, SLES)** – An ingredient added to soap to make it foamy. It's easily absorbed by the body and can lead to irritation of sensitive skin.

- **Triclosan** – Can be found in some hand sanitizers, deodorants, and antibacterial products. It has been linked to endocrine disorders and cancer.

- **Toluene** – Has been linked to endocrine and immune disorders. Often found in hair and nail products, this ingredient is often hidden under the term, "fragrance."

The All-Natural Ingredients You Can Use When Creating DIY Cosmetics

One of the great things about creating your own makeup is that you have total control over the ingredients you're going to use. In addition, gone are the days when sourcing hard to find ingredients seemed like an impossible task; nowadays, we can do a quick online search and find just about anything we want within a matter of seconds thanks to the power of almighty Google!

I admit that I wasn't exactly too crazy about making my own makeup in the beginning. It seemed like it required too much effort. But all of that changed when I started doing my own research on the ingredients other people were using to create their makeup. I was so impressed with the benefits that these ingredients provided that I had to try it out myself.

If you're feeling a bit overwhelmed by the idea of creating your own handmade makeup, don't be. Once you get to know your ingredients better, you will be more than happy to make the transition.

Here are just some of the all-natural ingredients you can incorporate in making your own line of all-natural DIY cosmetics.

- *Aloe Vera* - Aloe vera is packed with vitamins and minerals that don't just heal skin, they also lock in moisture. This gel-like substance is great for soothing and cooling skin, making it especially useful after a day in the sun! It's no wonder that Cleopatra is said to have used this miracle of nature as one of her go-to beauty regimen ingredients.

- *Cocoa Butter* - The same plant that gives us one of the best things ever, (chocolate!) also provides us with a skin softener like no other! Cocoa butter, which is rich in fatty acids, doesn't just smooth the skin, it also fights signs of aging. Whether you're trying to prevent wrinkles or you just want to give your skin a healthy treat, cocoa butter can do wonders in helping your skin stay soft and supple. A natural source of vitamin E, cocoa butter makes for the perfect moisturizer if used sparingly.

- *Coconut Oil* - One great thing about coconut oil is that it's safe to use on all skin types. Whether you're dealing with sensitive skin or you're one of the lucky ones who's blessed with problem-free skin, coconut oil makes a great all-around moisturizer.

- ***Jojoba Oil*** - Even though jojoba oil needs to be extracted from a dry desert shrub, it's a highly effective, all-natural moisturizers. Native Americans even used this miraculous oil in their traditional medicinal practices. In modern times, jojoba oil has become a crucial ingredient in many anti-aging products available on the market. Not only does it help reduce wrinkles, it can also help keep your skin looking clear and luminous.

- ***Lavender*** - This sweet-smelling flower, which is often used to treat anxiety and insomnia, also has a lesser-known beneficial property; the promotion of healthy cell turnover. As proof of its healing properties, ancient Romans used to wash injuries with lavender water. No wonder lavender is being touted as an herbal workhorse, helping to cure everything from hair loss to skin rashes!

- ***Olive Oil*** - We've all heard about the amazing effects this oil can have on the body when incorporated into a healthy diet. Olive oil is rich in antioxidants and vitamin E, which can help repair cell damage and fight free radicals. But olive oil isn't just great for skin care; it can also be a fantastic addition to your hair care routine. Just apply a little onto a dry scalp, leave overnight, and you're guaranteed to wake up with healthier looking hair the next day. (For more on natural homemade shampoos, check out the book, "Homemade Shampoo: A Complete Beginner's Guide to Natural DIY Shampoos You Can Make Today", by me, Jane Aniston. Click HERE to check it out!)

- **Shea Butter** - Shea butter's texture may seem a little overly-rich for cosmetics, but it's texture is what makes it another of the best all-natural moisturizers available. Shea butter can penetrate deep into the skin, stimulating cell regeneration. It doesn't just help to retain elasticity; it also promotes a healthy radiance that comes from within. High quality Shea butter can be a little pricey compared to some of the other ingredients mentioned in this book, but once you start to notice the results, you'll be happy you spent the few extra dollars and gave it a go!

- **Sunflower Oil** - Sunflower oil is a natural oil that's packed with easily absorbable vitamin E. As a natural emollient, it helps soften and nurture skin without having the heavy feel of a cream. Sunflower oil is also known to help stubborn scars to fade over time, making it a great oil to add to face creams and concealers.

- **Tea Tree Oil** - You're probably well aware that tea tree oil is the number one natural acne fighter, but did you know that it's also one of the strongest all-natural antiseptics around? As an antibacterial agent, it acts like an all-purpose germ killer that can be used to treat anything from small insect bites to wounds. Some studies even show that it's more powerful than benzoyl peroxide in treating acne!

Switching to Homemade Makeup

I hope this chapter has given you some insight into exactly why you should give homemade cosmetics a try, both in terms of the harmful chemicals they will allow you to avoid and the benefits which can be gained from using natural alternatives.

Switching to homemade makeup may take some getting used to, especially if you've been using designer/branded department store makeup for many years. Your skin may require some time to readjust itself to your new routine and there's the possibility of a few minor breakouts here and there.

One thing that really helped me with the transition was a good skin purifying regimen. I scouted around for the safest and most effective skin cleanser to make sure that my skin was not just clean, but also well nourished. If this is something you're not yet doing, I highly recommend you start, whether you decide to give homemade cosmetics a try or not.

With that said, we're almost ready to move on to the recipes, but before we do, I'll share with you my DIY makeup insider secrets! Make sure you read through the next chapter carefully before moving on to the recipes. If you do you'll be well-prepared and ready to start on whipping up your first batch of chemical-free cosmetics!

Chapter 2

Insider Tips On Creating Your Own Cosmetics

Creating your own makeup can be quite an experience. Not only do you get to create something amazing for your skin, but you also have the opportunity to learn more about how different ingredients can give you a healthy and natural flush of color without the need for expensive cosmetic products.

It doesn't matter where you got your inspiration from, the important thing is that you've taken that first step to a much healthier, natural makeup habit. Making your own cosmetic products will be a lot of fun, but there are some things you should be aware of before you begin. So before you grab that mixing bowl, here are a few insider tips to get you off to a good start and help you avoid any problems further down the road.

Prep your workspace

The first thing you need to do before you get started on your cosmetic creations is to prep your workspace.

Making your own makeup at home can get quite messy, so make sure that you have prepared a dedicated space for it which will be easy to clean up when you've finished. Working in the kitchen is perfectly fine, but if you're going to turn it into a habit, you might want to look around your home for a small area you can dedicate to makeup creation, space permitting of course.

Source your ingredients from a reliable supplier

Most of the ingredients needed to make your own homemade makeup can easily be bought from grocery stores. However, if you're looking for an ingredient that can't be easily purchased in your area, you can always find a reliable supplier online with a little searching. When sourcing ingredients, make sure to choose a supplier that is known first and foremost for their quality, and not just the quantity of product they are offering. Don't be fooled by a cheap price tag if you're not sure about the quality of the product. Think of these ingredients as you would food; they will be entering your body through your skin, so chose the best you can find or that you can afford.

Be aware of your allergies

Just because an ingredient is considered all-natural or organic doesn't mean that it's guaranteed to be 100% safe for you. It may work wonders for others, but there is the odd chance that for you it could cause an allergic reaction. So before you get started on any homemade makeup batches, make sure that the ingredients you're going to use are safe for you. Try to figure out which (if any) of the common ingredients may cause skin irritation. If you're going to work with an unfamiliar ingredient, test it first on your wrist to see if it causes a negative reaction. This way, you don't end up harming your skin in your quest for healthier makeup alternatives.

Start with small batches

Since your homemade makeup doesn't contain any chemical ingredients designed to prolong its lifespan, it's best to only make small batches at a time. Most of the recipes for the DIY makeup in this book will last for a matter of weeks, depending on the product. Therefore, it's highly recommended that you don't make too much at one time. One option to make your homemade cosmetics last longer is to store them in the fridge. However, as making fresh batches is quick, easy and fun, creating more is unlikely to be a major inconvenience!

Always store homemade makeup in appropriate containers

Once you've made a fresh batch of DIY makeup, it's critical that you store it in an appropriate container. As I mentioned above, your homemade makeup won't contain any chemical preservatives to prevent bacterial growth, so always make it a point to use sterile containers. Look for containers with airtight lids so your product won't be exposed to air, humidity, germs, and bacteria. Although not essential, glass containers are a good option as glass is inert, meaning no chemicals will be able to leach into your makeup.

Don't get too hung up on following the recipes to the letter

The amounts of the ingredients you'll need may seem a little vague (for example "1/8 cup" or "¼ teaspoon") but don't get too hung up on being exact; just follow the instructions as best you can to begin with. Making your own cosmetics is a lot like cooking; over time you'll get used to the recipes and will be able to adjust them to suit your own needs and preferences.

Now that you're well prepared, let's get started on the recipes! Ive broken the recipes down into chapters based on type. Whereas in some of my other books I start with an introduction to the recipe and talk a little about the benefits of each ingredient, in this book I've simply gone straight to each recipe without the introduction. The reason for this is that cosmetics recipes are less about scents and fragrances than the products in the other books I've written (shampoos, lip balms, deodorants etc), and therefore I didn't feel it was necessary to introduce each individually. With that said, let's move onto the recipes. Good luck!

Chapter 3

Natural Makeup Recipes - Face

So you've decided you want to enjoy all the perks of good makeup but without having to worry about subjecting your face to the cocktail of chemicals found in store bought cosmetics every morning? Here are just a few tried and tested liquid and powder makeup recipes that will help you achieve the smooth and healthy complexion you're after.

In this chapter we'll cover recipes for various makeup bases, foundations (both powder and liquid), concealers, blushers, bronzers and finishing powders. The recipes are quick and easy and most importantly the ingredients are natural and you won't break the bank to pay for them!

Let's get started by taking a look at the makeup bases. Have fun!

— MAKEUP BASES —

1. *Simple Soothing Makeup Base*

Ingredients:

- 1/2 cup aloe vera gel
- 3 teaspoons coconut oil

Instructions:

1. Put the aloe vera gel into a small bowl.
2. Melt the coconut oil in a pan or in the microwave.
3. Mix the aloe vera gel and coconut oil together.
4. Store in an airtight, appropriately sized container. Refrigerate to extend the product life.

2. *Oil-Control Makeup Base*

Ingredients:

- 3 teaspoons aloe vera gel
- ¼ teaspoon kaolin clay
- ¼ teaspoon arrowroot powder

Instructions:

1. Combine the clay and arrowroot powder in a small bowl.
2. Add the aloe vera gel to the clay and arrowroot and mix well until the consistency is smooth.
3. Store in an appropriately sized, airtight container. Refrigerate to extend the product life.

— FOUNDATIONS —

3. *Powder Foundation for Normal Skin*

Ingredients:

- ¼ cup arrowroot powder
- Cinnamon powder

Instructions:

1. Place the arrowroot powder in a small container.
2. Add the cinnamon, bit by bit, until you achieve the right shade for your skin tone.
3. Store in an appropriately sized, airtight container.
4. Use a large powder brush for application.

4. *Powder Foundation for Dry Skin*

Ingredients:

- ¼ cup rice bran powder
- Cocoa powder

Instructions:

1. Place the rice bran powder into a small container.
2. Add the cocoa powder, bit by bit, until you achieve the right shade for your skin tone.
3. Store in an appropriately sized, airtight container.
4. Use a large powder brush for application.

5. Powder Foundation for Oily Skin

Ingredients:

- 1/8 cup arrowroot powder
- 1/8 cup green clay
- Nutmeg powder (amount depends on the shade you want to achieve)

Instructions:

1. Place the arrowroot powder and the green clay into a small container and mix together.
2. Add the nutmeg powder, bit by bit, until you achieve the desired shade for your skin tone.
3. Store in an appropriately sized, airtight container.
4. Use a large powder brush for application.

6. *Liquid Foundation for Normal Skin*

Ingredients:

- 3 tablespoons almond oil
- 2 tablespoons cocoa butter, melted
- 1 vitamin-E gel capsule
- Cocoa powder

Instructions:

1. Melt the cocoa butter in a microwave oven or by heating gently in a small pan on the stove.
2. Whisk the almond oil and the cocoa butter together in a small bowl.
3. Prick the vitamin-E gel capsule and squeeze the contents into the bowl containing the mixture.
4. Mix well until you achieve a smooth consistency.
5. Add the cocoa powder, 1/8 teaspoon at a time, until you get the color you desire. Make sure to whisk the mixture well each time you add more color.

6. Store in an appropriately sized, airtight container.

7. Liquid Foundation for Dry Skin

Ingredients:

- 3 tablespoons coconut oil
- 1 tablespoon Shea butter, melted
- 1 vitamin-E gel capsule
- Cocoa powder

Instructions:

1. Melt the coconut oil and the Shea butter in a microwave oven or by heating gently in a small pan on the stove.
2. Whisk the coconut oil and the Shea butter together in a small bowl.
3. Prick the vitamin-E gel capsule and squeeze the contents into the small bowl with the mixture.
4. Mix until you achieve a smooth consistency.
5. Add the cocoa powder, 1/8 teaspoon at a time, until you get the color you want. Make sure to whisk the mixture well each time you add more color.

6. Store in an appropriately sized, airtight container.

8. *Liquid Foundation for Oily Skin*

Ingredients:

- 3 tablespoons almond oil
- 1 tablespoon beeswax
- 1 vitamin-E gel capsule
- Cinnamon powder

Instructions:

1. Melt the beeswax in a microwave oven or by heating gently in a small pan on the stove.
2. Whisk the almond oil and the beeswax together in a small bowl.
3. Prick the vitamin-E gel capsule and add the contents to the mixture in the bowl.
4. Mix well until you achieve a smooth consistency.
5. Add the cinnamon powder, 1/8 teaspoon at a time, until you reach the desired shade. Make sure to whisk the mixture well each time you add more color.

6. Store in an appropriately sized, airtight container.

— CONCEALER —

9. *Blemish Control Concealer*

Ingredients:

- 1 tablespoon Shea butter, melted
- ½ teaspoon tea tree oil
- Cocoa powder
- Low-grade cinnamon powder

Instructions:

1. Melt the Shea butter in a microwave or by heating gently in a small pan on the stove.
2. Whisk the Shea butter and tea tree oil together in a small bowl.
3. Mix the cocoa powder and cinnamon powder in a separate bowl.
4. Add the cocoa powder and cinnamon powder mixture to the Shea butter and tea tree oil, 1/8 teaspoon at a time, until you get

the color you want. Make sure to whisk the mixture well each time you add color.

5. Store in an appropriately sized, airtight container.

— BLUSHERS —

10. *Simple Flush Blusher*

Ingredients:

- 1 tablespoon arrowroot powder
- Beet powder
- Low-grade cinnamon

Instructions:

1. Place the arrowroot powder in a small container.
2. Combine the beet powder and cinnamon powder in a separate bowl.
3. Add the beet powder/cinnamon mixture, 1 teaspoon at a time, until you get the color you want.
4. Mix well.
5. Store in an appropriately sized, airtight container.

6. Use a large powder brush for application.

11. Raspberry Crush Blusher

Ingredients:

- 1 tablespoon arrowroot powder
- Raspberry powder (from freeze-dried raspberries)

Instructions:

1. Place the arrowroot powder in a small container.
2. Use a coffee grinder to turn freeze-dried raspberries into a fine powder.
3. Add the raspberry powder, 1 teaspoon at a time, to the arrowroot powder, until you get the color you want.
4. Mix well.
5. Store in an appropriately sized, airtight container.
6. Use a large powder brush for application.

12. *Hibiscus Blusher*

Ingredients:

- 1 tablespoon arrowroot powder
- Hibiscus powder
- Low-grade cinnamon

Instructions:

1. Place the arrowroot powder in a small container.
2. In a separate bowl, mix the cinnamon powder and the hibiscus powder.
3. Add the hibiscus powder/cinnamon mixture, 1 teaspoon at a time, until you reach the desired shade.
4. Mix well.
5. Store in an appropriately sized, airtight container.
6. Use a large powder brush for application.

— BRONZERS —

13. *Contour Powder*

Ingredients:

- 2 teaspoon cornstarch
- 1 teaspoon nutmeg powder
- 1 teaspoon cocoa powder
- 1 tablespoon low-grade cinnamon powder
- 15 drops rosemary essential oil

Instructions:

1. Mix the nutmeg powder, cocoa powder, and cinnamon powder together with the cornstarch. Make sure that the combined powders are thoroughly mixed.
2. Add the rosemary essential oil to the powders, and again, mix thoroughly.
3. Break down any clumps that have form so the mixture is even.

4. Place the mixture into an empty compact and flatten down with a spatula or the back of a spoon.

5. Use a wedge sponge for a smooth and well-blended application.

14. Simple Bronzing Powder

Ingredients:

- 1 tablespoon cornstarch
- 2 tablespoons low-grade cinnamon powder

Instructions:

1. Simply combine the cornstarch and cinnamon powder in a small bowl and mix well.
2. Store in an appropriately sized, airtight container.
3. Use a large powder brush for application. Make sure to use sparingly so as to subtly enhance and contour the face. Adjust the composition of the mixture slightly to change the tone.

— FINISHING POWDERS —

15. *Silky Smooth Finishing Powder*

Ingredients:

- 1 tablespoon cornstarch
- Cocoa powder

Instructions:

1. Place the cornstarch into a small container
2. Add the cocoa powder, little by little, and mix. Keep adding the cocoa until you reach the desired shade.
3. Store in an appropriately sized, airtight container.
4. Use a large, soft brush when applying to the face.

16. Oil Control Finishing Powder

Ingredients:

- 1 tablespoon orris root powder
- Nutmeg powder

Instructions:

1. Place the orris root powder into a small container.
2. Add nutmeg powder, little by little, and mix. Keep adding the nutmeg until you get the shade you want.
3. Store in an appropriately sized, airtight container.
4. Use a large, soft brush when applying to the face.

Chapter 4

Natural Makeup Recipes – Eyes

When it comes to the skin around your eyes, you should be especially concerned about avoiding the chemical nasties used in so many cosmetic products, as the skin here is more delicate and susceptible to damage than most. Not only that, but our eyes are also one of the first areas that start to wrinkle and show signs of aging.

In this chapter we'll take a look at some eye shadows, eye liners and mascaras. If you want to emphasize your eyes without running the risk of damaging the skin around them, give these recipes a try.

— EYE SHADOWS —

17. *Cream Eye Shadow*

Base Ingredients:

- 1 tablespoon arrowroot powder
- 1 tablespoon Shea butter, melted

Colorant Ingredients:

- Cocoa powder
- Cinnamon powder
- Nutmeg
- Beet powder
- Allspice
- Turmeric
- Spirulina

Instructions:

1. Place the arrowroot powder in a small bowl.

2. Choose your preferred colorant ingredient/s based on the color you desire.

3. Combine and mix until you get your desired shade. Have fun experimenting with different color combinations.

4. Add the melted Shea butter, ¼ teaspoon at a time, and mix thoroughly until you reach a thick, creamy consistency.

5. Transfer the cream eye shadow mixture to an appropriately sized, airtight container and use as you would a regular eye shadow.

18. *Powder Eye shadow*

Base Ingredient:

- 1 tablespoon rice powder

Colorant Ingredients:

- Cocoa powder
- Cinnamon powder
- Nutmeg
- Beet powder
- Allspice
- Turmeric
- Spirulina

Instructions:

1. Place the rice powder into a small bowl.
2. Choose your preferred colorant ingredient/s based on the color you desire.

3. Combine and mix until you get your desired shade. Have fun experimenting with different color combinations.

4. Transfer the powder eye shadow to an appropriately sized, airtight container.

— EYE LINERS —

19. *Natural Cream Eyeliner (Black)*

Ingredients:

- 4 capsules activated charcoal
- Few drops olive oil

Instructions:

1. Place the activated charcoal in a small bowl.
2. Add the olive oil, 1 drop at a time (mixing as you do), until you produce a smooth creamy texture.
3. Store in an appropriately sized, airtight container.

20. Natural Cream Eyeliner (Brown)

Ingredients:

- 1 tablespoon cocoa powder
- Few drops olive oil

Instructions:

1. Place the cocoa powder into a small bowl.
2. Add the olive oil, 1 drop at a time, until you get a smooth creamy texture.
3. Store in an appropriately sized, airtight container.

— MASCARAS —

21. *Natural Mascara (Black)*

Ingredients:

- 2 capsules activated charcoal
- 2 teaspoons coconut oil, melted
- 1 teaspoon beeswax, melted
- 4 teaspoons aloe vera gel

Instructions:

1. Place the activated charcoal into a small bowl.
2. Add the coconut oil, beeswax, and aloe vera gel. Make sure you blend well until the mixture holds.
3. Transfer the mixture to a cleaned, used mascara container.

22. *Natural Mascara (Brown)*

Ingredients:

- 1 tablespoon cocoa powder
- 2 teaspoons coconut oil, melted
- 1 teaspoon beeswax, melted
- 4 teaspoons aloe vera gel

Instructions:

1. Place the cocoa powder into a small bowl.
2. Add the coconut oil, beeswax, and aloe vera gel. Make sure to blend well until the mixture holds.
3. Transfer the mixture to a cleaned, used mascara container.

Chapter 5
Natural Makeup Recipes – Lips

Studies have shown that there are still lipsticks out on the market that contain small amounts of lead. Lead can be, as you probably already know, extremely damaging to human health.

If you want to pamper your lips with all-natural alternatives and avoid the risk of potentially introducing toxins to your body, follow the simple recipes in this chapter. Another great thing about making your own homemade lippie is that you can easily customize the color and consistency by tweaking just a few key ingredients!

In this chapter we'll start by covering easy-glide lipsticks, then we'll take a look at matte lipsticks before finally moving on to the glossy lipsticks.

— EASY-GLIDE LIPSTICKS —

23. *Easy Glide Lipstick (Red)*

Ingredients:

- 1 teaspoon cocoa butter
- 1 teaspoon beeswax pastilles
- Beetroot powder

Instructions:

1. Melt the cocoa butter and the beeswax in a small microwavable bowl.
2. Add the beetroot powder, 1/8 teaspoon at a time, until you get the shade you desire. If you want a clear gloss, this can be achieved with around 1/8 teaspoon, while ¼ teaspoon will produce a slightly stronger shade.
3. Store in an appropriately sized, airtight container and apply with your finger as you would a lip gloss.

24. *Easy Glide Lipstick (Nude)*

Ingredients:

- 1 teaspoon cocoa butter
- 1 teaspoon beeswax pastilles
- 1 teaspoon coconut oil
- Cocoa powder

Instructions:

1. Melt the cocoa butter, beeswax, and coconut oil in a small microwavable bowl.
2. Add the cocoa powder, 1/8 teaspoon at a time, until you get the shade you want. You can achieve a clear gloss with 1/8 teaspoon, while ¼ teaspoon will produce a slightly stronger shade.
3. Store in an appropriately sized, airtight container and apply with your finger as you would a lip gloss.

— MATTE LIPSTICKS —

25. Matte Lipstick (Red)

Ingredients:

- 1 teaspoon cocoa butter
- 1 teaspoon beeswax pastilles
- ¼ teaspoon bentonite clay
- Beetroot powder

Instructions:

1. Melt the cocoa butter and the beeswax in in a small microwavable bowl.
2. Add the bentonite clay to the mix.
3. Add the beet root powder, 1/8 teaspoon at a time, until you achieve the desired shade.
4. Store in an appropriately sized, airtight container and apply with your finger as you would a lip gloss.

26. Matte Lipstick (Tan)

Ingredients:

- 1 teaspoon cocoa butter
- 1 teaspoon beeswax pastilles
- ¼ teaspoon bentonite clay
- Cocoa powder

Instructions:

1. Melt the cocoa butter and beeswax in a small microwavable bowl.
2. Add the bentonite clay to the mix.
3. Add the cocoa powder, 1/8 teaspoon at a time, until you get the shade you want.
4. Store in an appropriately sized, airtight container and apply with your finger as you would a lip gloss.

— GLOSSY LIPSTICKS —

27. Glossy Lipstick (Red)

Ingredients:

- 1 teaspoon cocoa butter
- 1 teaspoon beeswax pastilles
- 1 teaspoon olive oil
- Beetroot powder

Instructions:

1. Melt the cocoa butter, beeswax, and olive oil in a small microwavable bowl.
2. Add the beetroot powder, 1/8 teaspoon at a time, until you get the desired shade. You can achieve a clear gloss with about 1/8 teaspoon, while ¼ teaspoon will produce a stronger shade.
3. Store in an appropriately sized, airtight container and apply with your finger as you would a lip gloss.

28. Glossy Lipstick (Nude)

Ingredients:

- 1 teaspoon cocoa butter
- 1 teaspoon beeswax pastilles
- 1 teaspoon olive oil
- Cocoa powder

Instructions:

1. Melt the cocoa butter, beeswax, and olive oil in a small microwavable bowl.
2. You can achieve a clear gloss with about 1/8 teaspoon, while ¼ teaspoon will produce a stronger shade.
3. Store in an appropriately sized, airtight container and apply with your finger as you would a lip gloss.

Conclusion

The way we choose to spend our money is important. If we continue to support companies that make a profit from endangering our health, it could be said that we are exercising poor judgment and failing to act wisely.

I believe it's important that we each do our own research into the cosmetics we buy and use. For our health's sake, as well as the health of others who use these products, it pays to be an informed consumer and to vote with our dollars.

Thank you again for downloading this book. I hope you enjoyed reading it and were able to learn a lot about the benefits of making your own makeup at home. What's more, I hope you will actually try some of the recipes for yourself and that you're able to experience the benefits of using these natural, healthy alternatives to store-bought cosmetics!

A message from the author, Jane Aniston

Finally, if you enjoyed this book, **please** take the time to post a review on Amazon. It will only take a couple of minutes and I'd be extremely grateful for your support. Thank you.

Jane Aniston

FREE BONUS!: Preview Of "Homemade Shampoo - A Complete Beginner's Guide to Natural DIY Shampoos You Can Make Today" - Includes 34 Organic Shampoo Recipes!'

If you enjoyed this book, I have a little bonus for you! This is a preview of one of my other books "Homemade Shampoo - A Complete Beginner's Guide to Natural DIY Shampoos You Can Make Today", which exposes the secrets of the hidden toxins lurking in your store-bought shampoos! This book also includes 34 simple and enjoyable organic shampoo recipes that you can make at home today. Keep your hair beautiful without exposing yourself to potentially harmful chemical nasties! Enjoy!

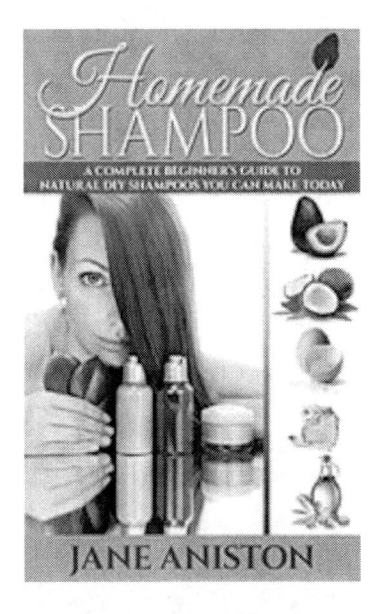

Chapter 1: Why You Should Stop Using Store-bought Shampoos and Start Making Your Own Natural Shampoos at Home!

There are hundreds of shampoos on the market and each one of them promises to leave your hair shinier, softer and more beautiful than the rest. Realistically though, these shampoos rarely live up to their lofty promises, and in fact, for a number of reasons that we'll go into in this book, by far the best option is to simply make your own natural shampoos at home.

While the vast majority of us grow up believing that using store-bought shampoos is the only option, it's never too late to understand that there is actually a better alternative. After looking more carefully at what's actually in most store-bought shampoos, I highly recommend you give making your own toxin-free, natural homemade shampoos a try, as these products are far better for your hair, your health, and the environment.

You're probably wondering why you should spend the extra time and energy to make your own shampoos when you can easily grab a bottle off the shelf in your local supermarket? Well, here's a rundown of facts that will help you understand why homemade shampoos are most definitely better than the store-bought variety!

1. **Natural homemade shampoos take fantastic care of your hair.** Contrary to popular belief, it isn't necessary to wash our hair with chemical shampoo every day. The reason for this is that over-shampooing strips the hair of it's natural oils, and due to their harshness, this is particularly true of store-bought shampoos. However, when you begin using homemade shampoos you'll notice that your hair will look healthier and that the right amount of protective natural oils will remain intact.

2. **You can make natural homemade shampoos in small amounts and keep them in non-polluting, reusable containers until you need them.** Most of the shampoos in this book can be stored in the fridge for at least a few days, and up to a couple of weeks, saving you from having to regularly make new batches. Although a regular shampoo container can be used to store your homemade shampoos, the best way of storing them is in glass containers. The reason for this is that glass is inert meaning no chemicals can

leach out into your shampoos. As these containers are reusable and made of non-toxic material you'll also have the peace of mind that you're not just doing what's right for your hair, but also what's right for the environment!

3. **Store-bought shampoos are often full of potentially cancer-causing chemicals.** As we are all well aware, cancer is a truly awful disease! Therefore it's important that we do whatever we can in order to reduce the risk of ever suffering from this terrible condition. Cocamide DEA, a chemical found in nearly a hundred types of store-bought shampoos in the USA, has a proven link to the formation of cancerous cells in humans. Most shampoos also contain vast amounts of sulfates and parabens that may poison the scalp and the kidneys, and could also play a part in the onset of allergies. When you're using store-bought shampoos, you're exposing yourself to a vast array of chemical nasties, and in so doing you're putting yourself at risk of potentially damaging your body's tissues and organs. Other chemicals to beware of include:

- **Formaldehyde.** Yes, that's the same formaldehyde used for embalming the dead! While it may be OK for the dead, it's certainly not something we want to be introducing into our bodies while we're still alive! Formaldehyde can play a part in cancer formation and can reportedly cause our body's organs to stiffen. This in turn may contribute to the onset of organ damage.

- **Sodium Laureth Sulphate.** This chemical slowly damages the hair by breaking down it's natural protein structure. An additional downside is that it can in some cases lead to lung or eye irritation.

- **Polyoxyethylene, Sodium Chloride, and other Thickening Agents.** These chemical agents are used to help shampoo lather easily. However, they can actually cause your scalp to become dry and itchy as they remove the natural oils which work to keep the hair and scalp healthy.

- **Synthetic Colors.** These chemicals can cause irritation of the scalp and skin.

- **Siloxane, Dimethicone, Silicone and other Hair Sealants.** These ingredients are reported to make the hair shiny, but due to their harsh chemical nature they can actually prevent the scalp from being able to coat hair with it's natural oils. This in turn can lead to dry, frizzy and hard-to-manage hair.

- **Mineral Oil, Petroleum, and Lanolin.** While these products claim to moisturize your hair, they actually have no proven benefits. Like most chemicals in commercially available shampoos, they can strip away the natural oils and moisture from the hair and in extreme cases may even cause the hair to thin or, at worst, fall out!

- **Propylene Glycol or Anti-Freeze Agents.** You may be wondering (as I was when I first found out), "Why on earth would there be anti-freeze in my shampoo!?" Well, quite simply it's used in order to stop the shampoo from freezing while in transport. This is the same anti-freeze that you might use in your car and, needless to say, it's NOT something that you want to be rubbing into your scalp! Anti-freezing agents may cause allergic reactions as well as skin irritation.

- **Alcohol.** The relatively high amounts of alcohol found in some of the shampoos available on store shelves may dry the hair and make it heavy and brittle.

As you can see, there are a wide range of potentially harmful ingredients in some store-bought shampoos. If we really care about the health of our hair and our bodies, perhaps we should think twice about using them and give alternative options a chance.

Check out the rest of "Homemade Shampoo: A Complete Beginner's Guide To Natural DIY Shampoos You Can Make Today" by Jane Aniston on Amazon.

Check Out My Other Books!

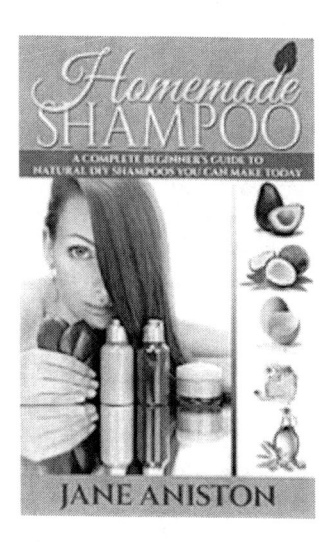

Homemade Shampoo (Includes 34 Organic Shampoo Recipes!)

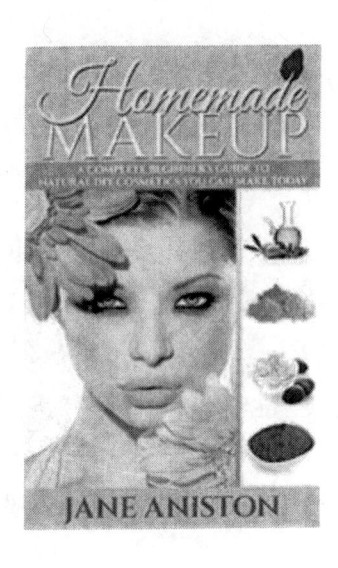

Homemade Makeup (Includes 28 Organic Makeup Recipes!)

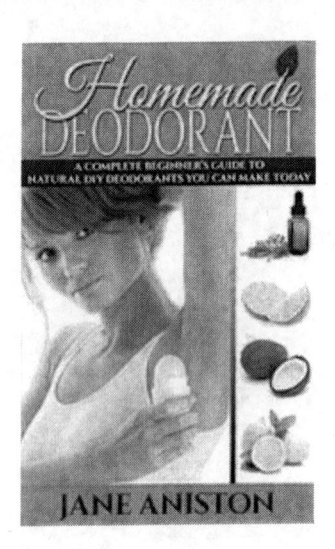

Homemade Deodorant (Includes 20 Organic Deodorant Recipes!)

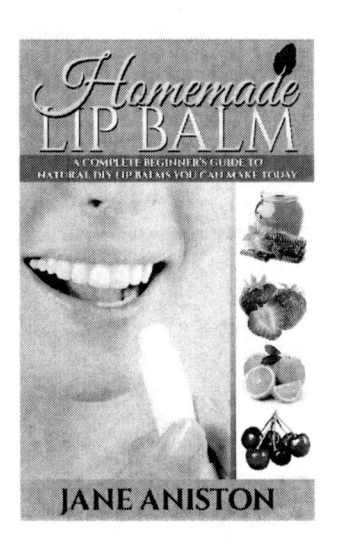

Homemade Lip Balm (Includes 22 Organic Lip Balm Recipes!)

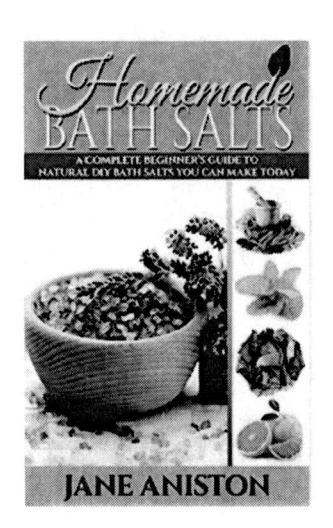

Homemade Bath Salts (Includes 35 Organic Bath Salt Recipes!)